JOSEPH SUSTE
WEANING A NATURAL STEP

A Gentle Nudge in Story Form

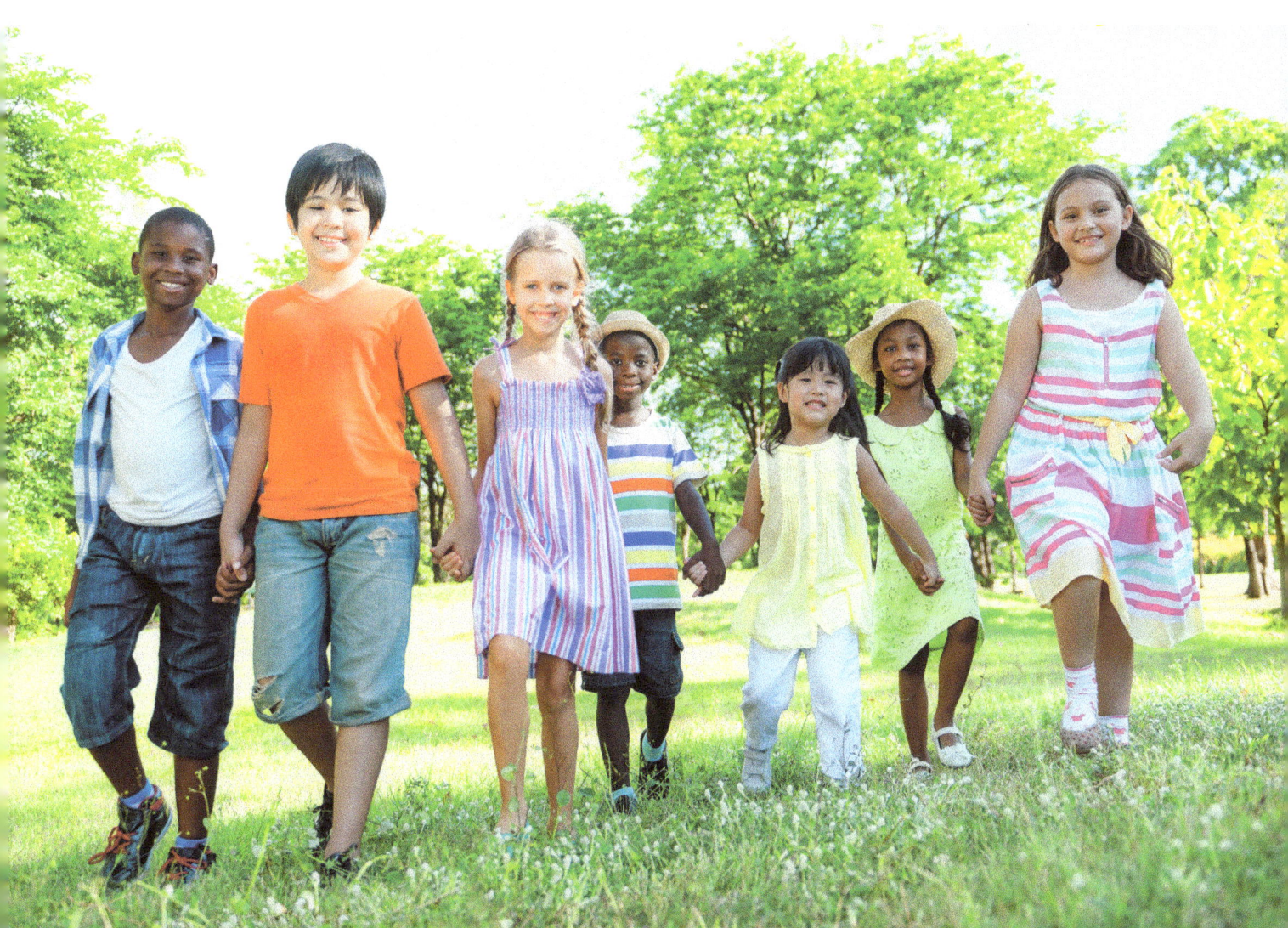

WEANING
A NATURAL STEP

JOSEPH SUSTE

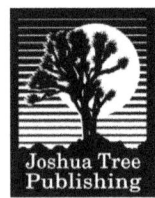

JoshuaTreePublishing.com
• *Chicago* •

ISBN 13-Digit: 978-1-941049-81-5

Copyright © 2019 Joseph Suste All Rights Reserved.

All rights reserved. No part of this book may be reproduced or transmitted in any form or by any means, electronic or mechanical, including information storage and retrieval system without written permission from the publisher, except by a reviewer who may quote brief passages in a review.

Original Illustration Copyrights:
Front Cover: ©Anna Om; **Back Cover**: ©Monkey Business;
p. 1, 28 © Photomorphic PTE. Ltd; p.3 © Sergey Novikov (serrnovik) ripicts.com;
p. 4, 5, 7, 28 © 2002lubava1981; p. 8 ©sdbower; p. 9, 28 © Vladimir Wrangel; p. 11, 28 © kamira;
p. 12 ©Tim W; p. 13, 28 © calypso137; p. 14 ©natasnow; p. 15, 28 © Blair Howard;
p. 17, 28 © gekaskr; p. 18 ©denisval p. 19, 28 © Nataliya Dvukhimenna; p. 20 ©gilitukha;
p. 21, 28 © arkady_z; p. 22 ©Bruder; p. 23, 28 © Vera Kuttelvaserova; p. 24 ©natasnow;
p. 25, 28 © virsuziglis; p. 27, 28 © micromonkey; p. 29 ©drubig-photo

Disclaimer:
This book is designed to provide information about the subject matter covered. The opinions expressed in this book are those of the author, not the publisher. Every effort has been made to make this book as complete and as accurate as possible. However, there may be mistakes both typographical and in content. Therefore, this text should be used only as a general guide and not as the ultimate source of information. The author and publisher of this book shall have neither liability nor responsibility to any person or entity with respect to any loss or damage caused or alleged to be caused directly or indirectly by the information contained in this book.

Printed in the United States of America

A note from the author

This writing takes me back to the 4th or 5th year of my childhood and a sweet memory of my mother nursing my newborn baby sister early one morning, while my brother, my three sisters, and I gathered around them, excited with the new member of our family. It was a joyful experience for all of us which I will never forget.

Joseph Suste

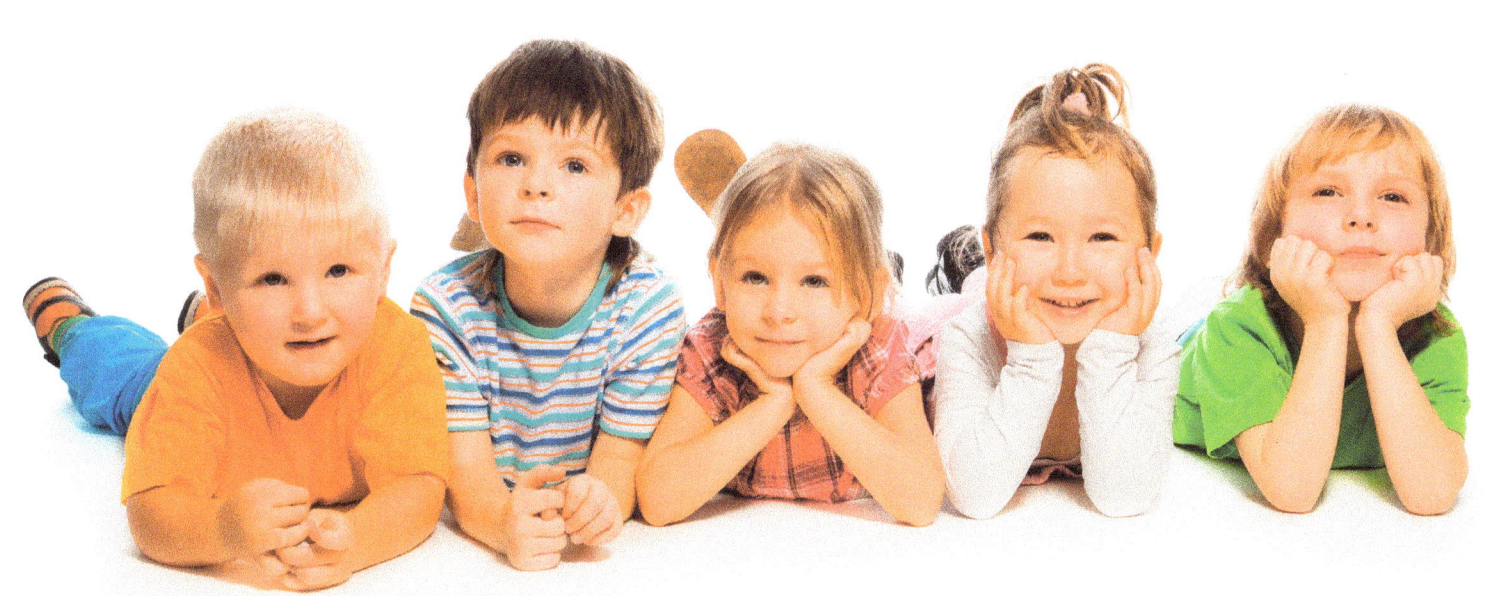

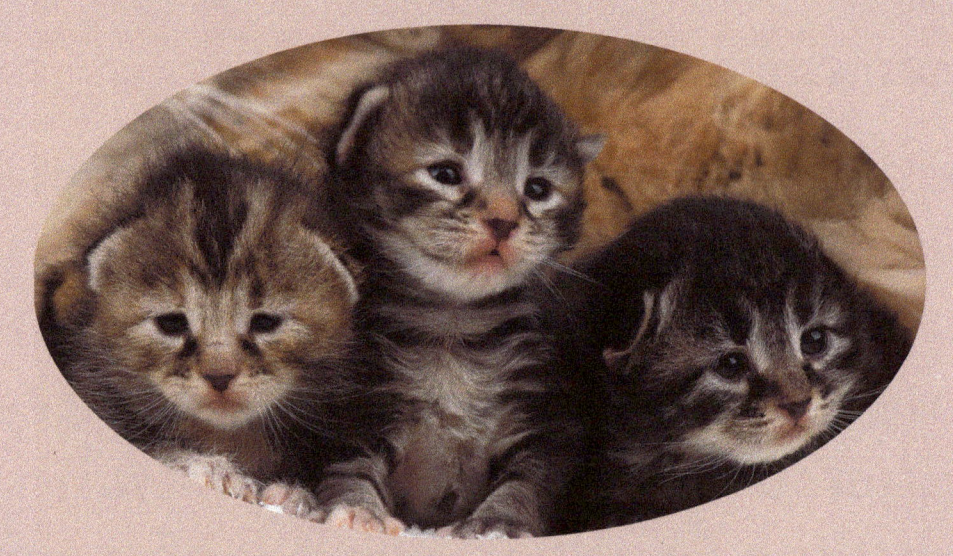

When this little kitten was born, he couldn't see, and he could barely walk. His momma had to do everything for him.
He couldn't eat the food grown-up cats eat.

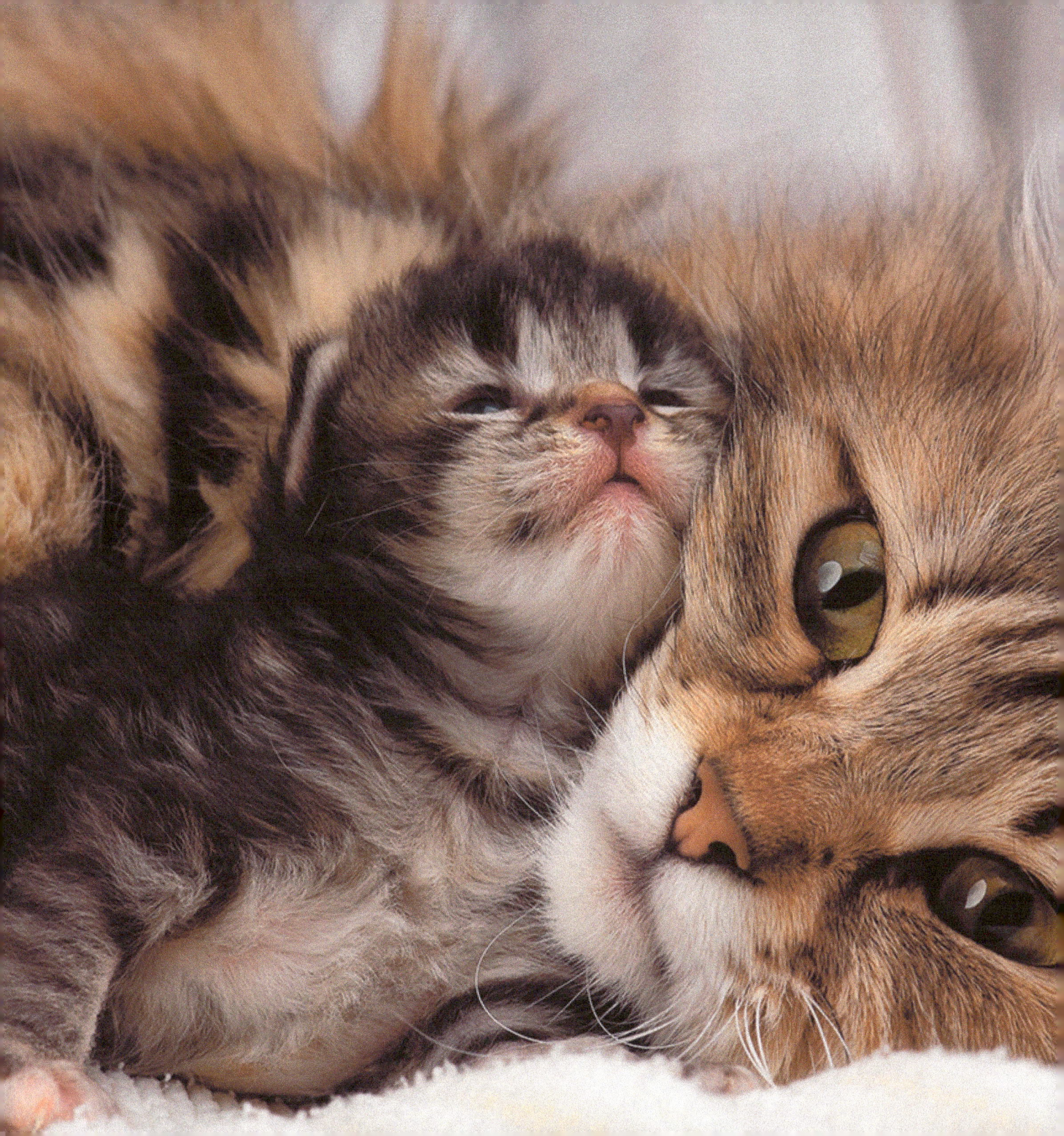

Lucky for him, his momma cat has lots of milk.

His mother's milk has everything a cuddly kitten needs to grow strong.

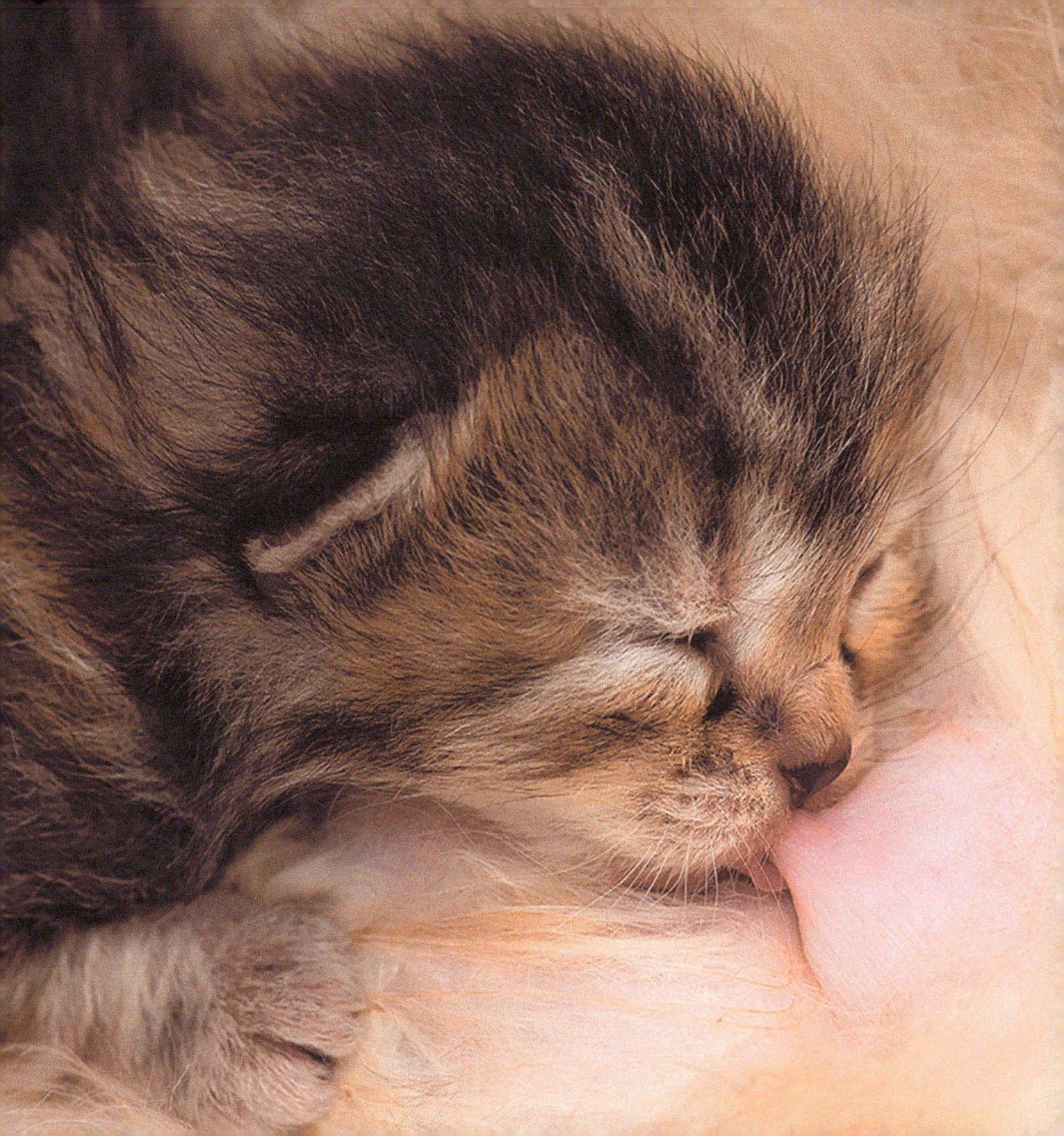

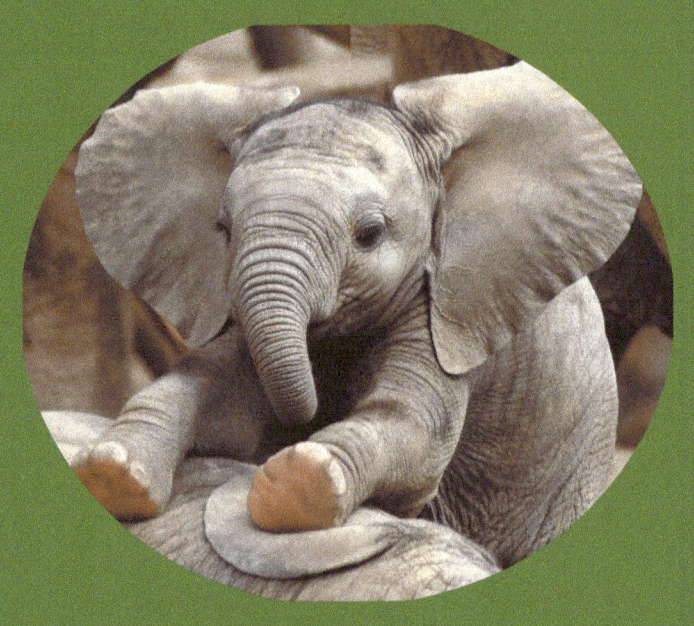

Many babies need milk from their mother right after they are born.

This momma elephant's milk is perfect for her baby girl.

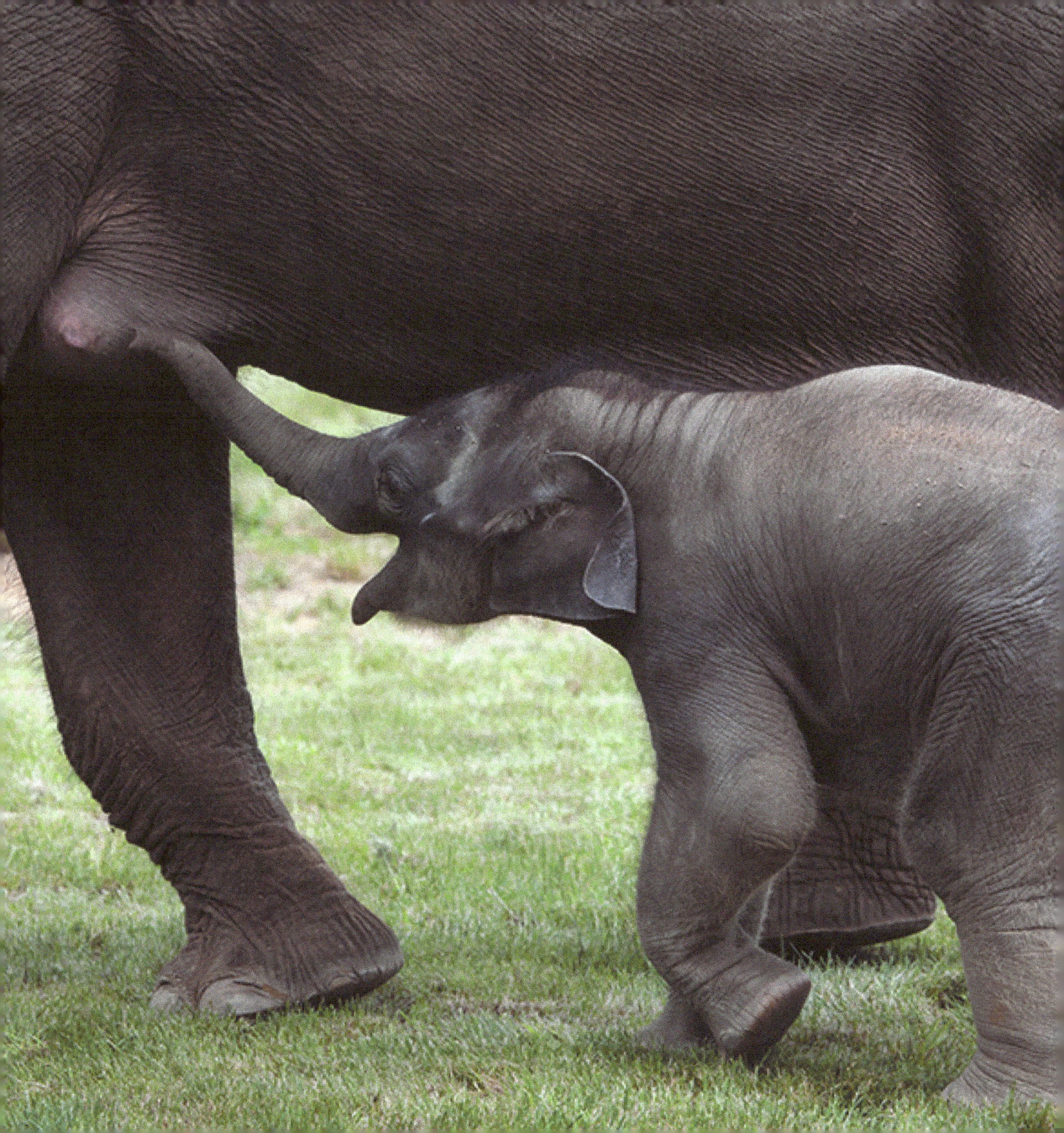

This little guy can't even stand up yet.

He's going to need his momma to feed him milk right away.

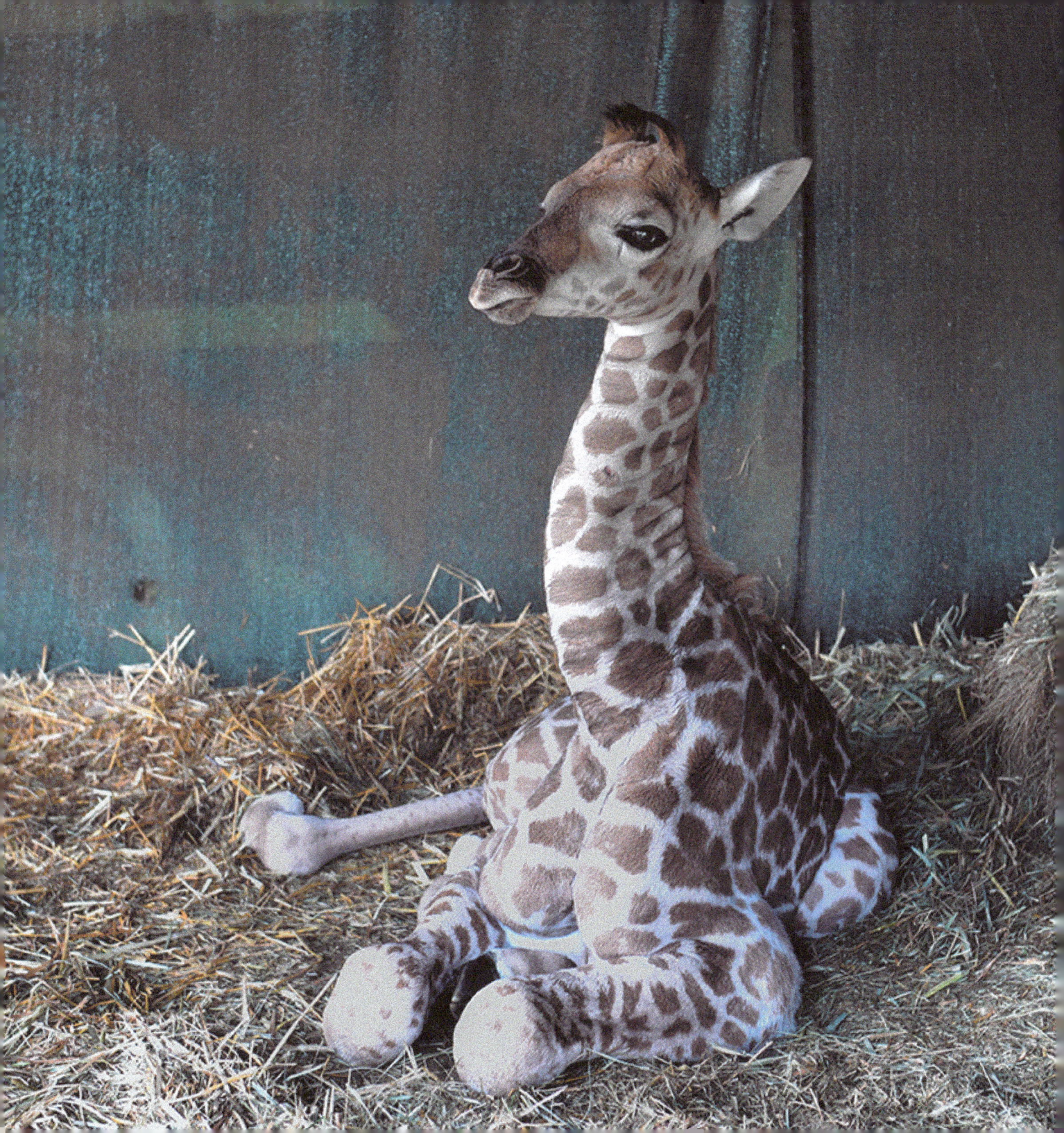

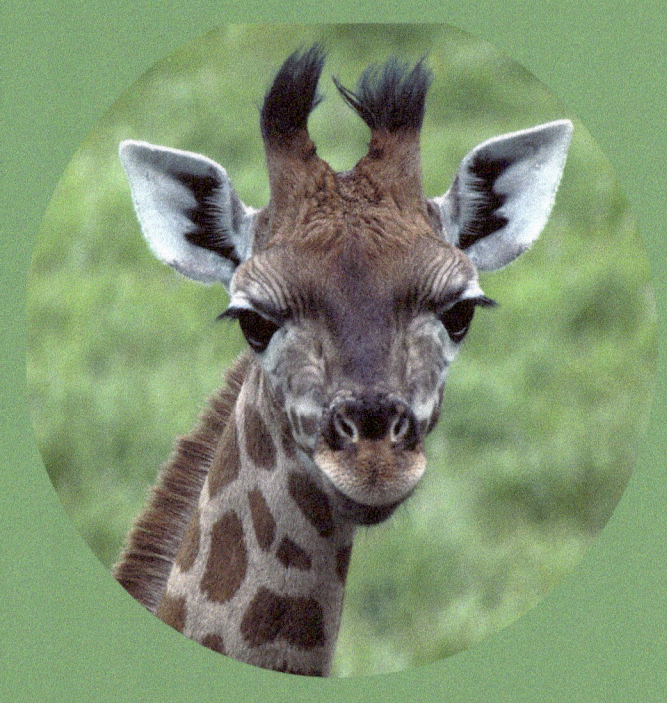

When momma's milk makes his legs strong, he can stand to nurse.

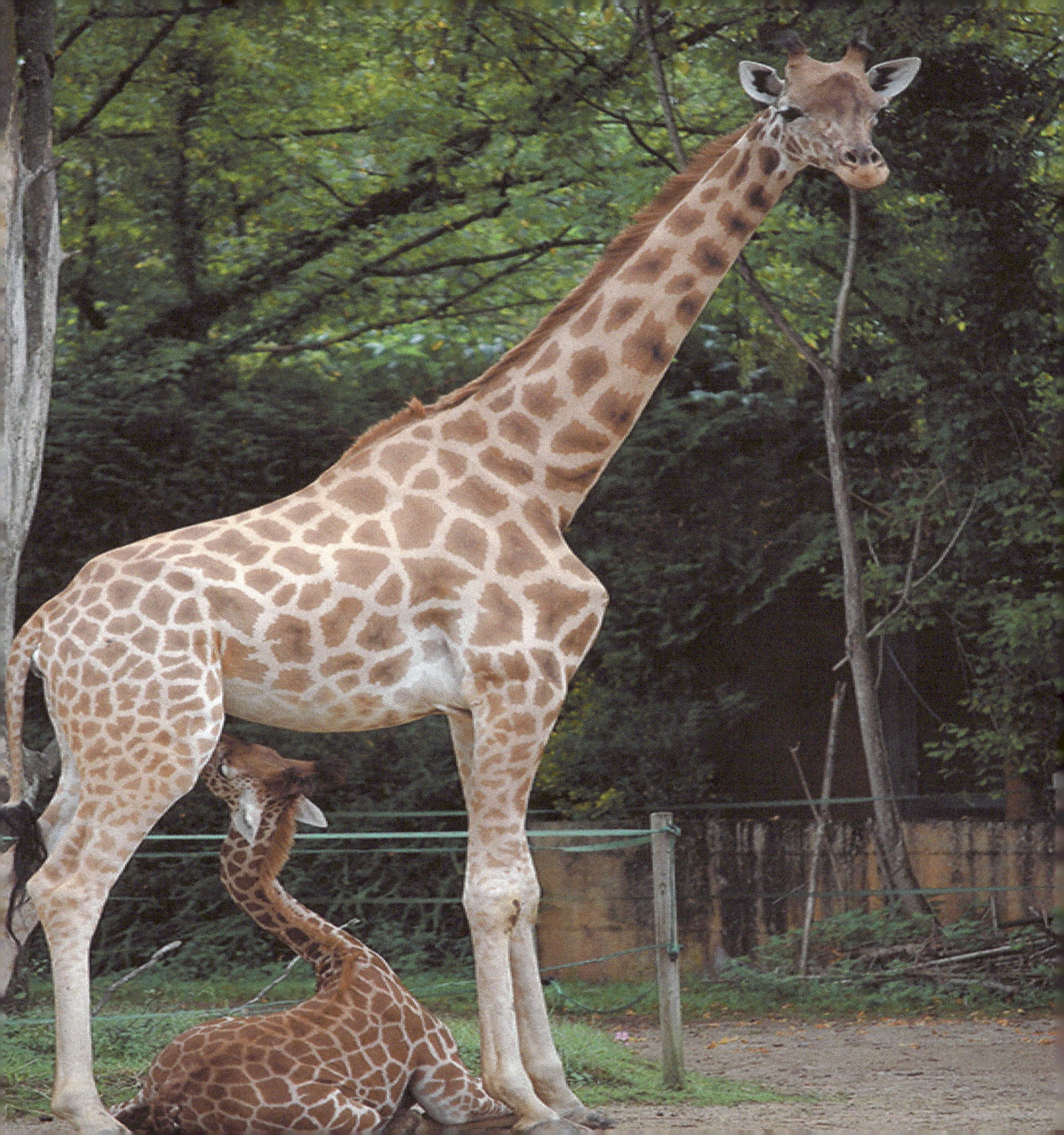

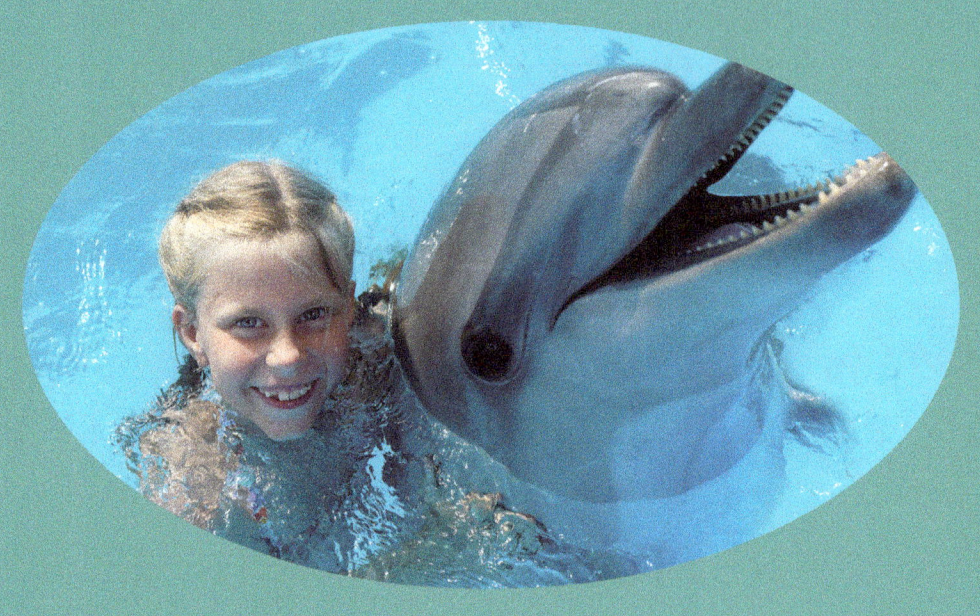

Even baby dolphins get milk from their mothers right after they are born.

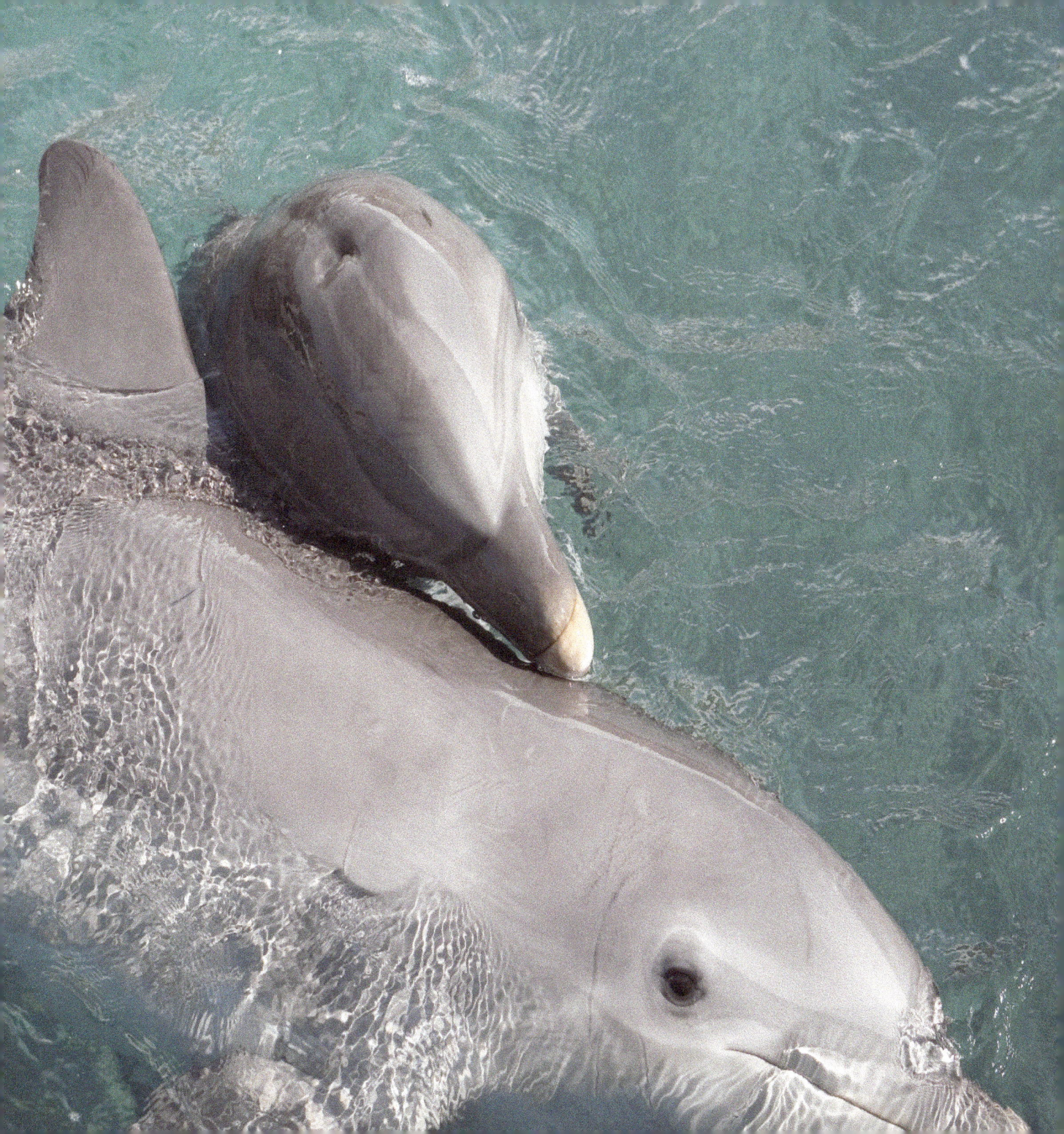

And look! Other babies need milk from their mothers! Girls and boys can't eat grown-up food when they are born either. They need mother's milk, too.

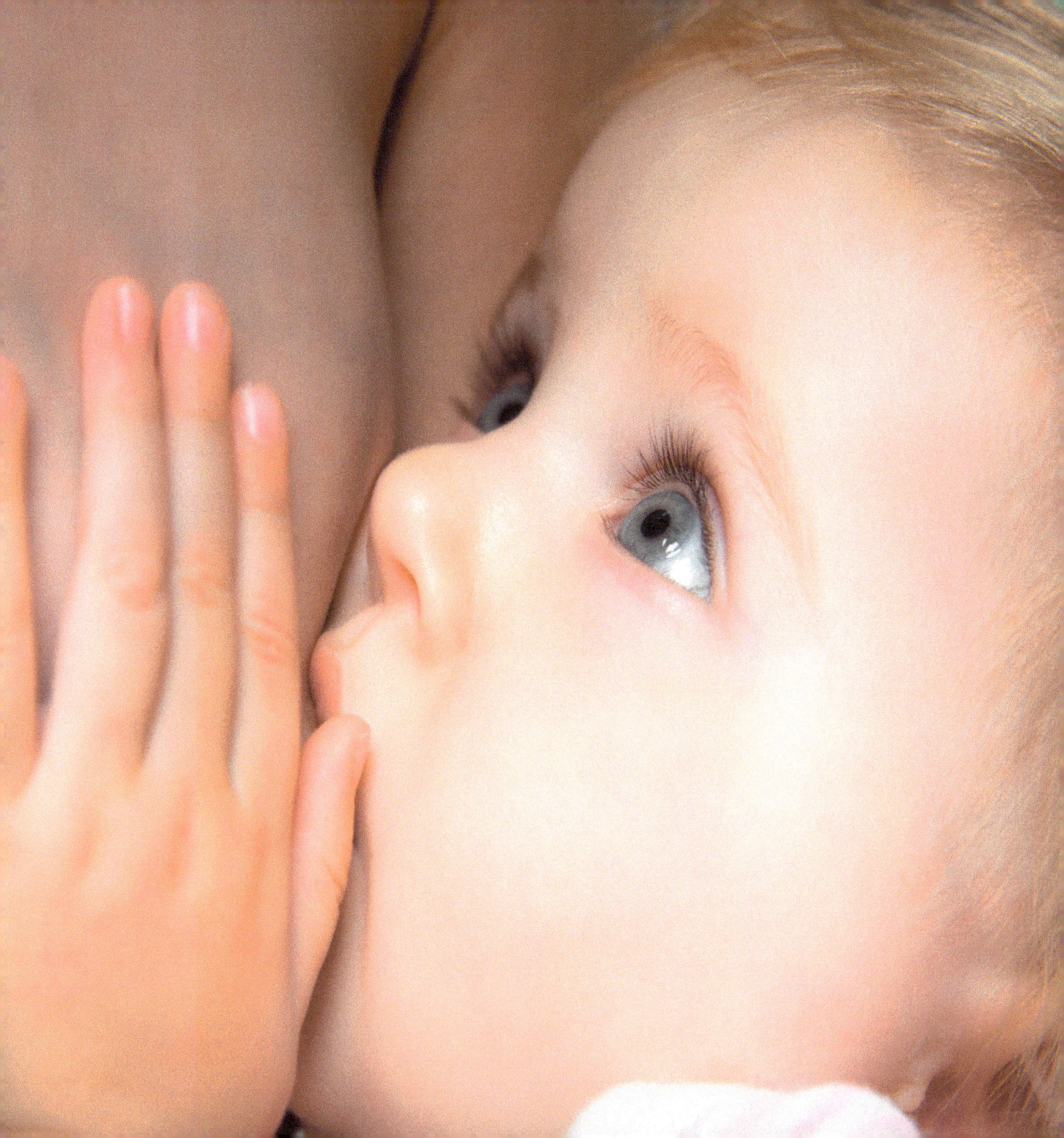

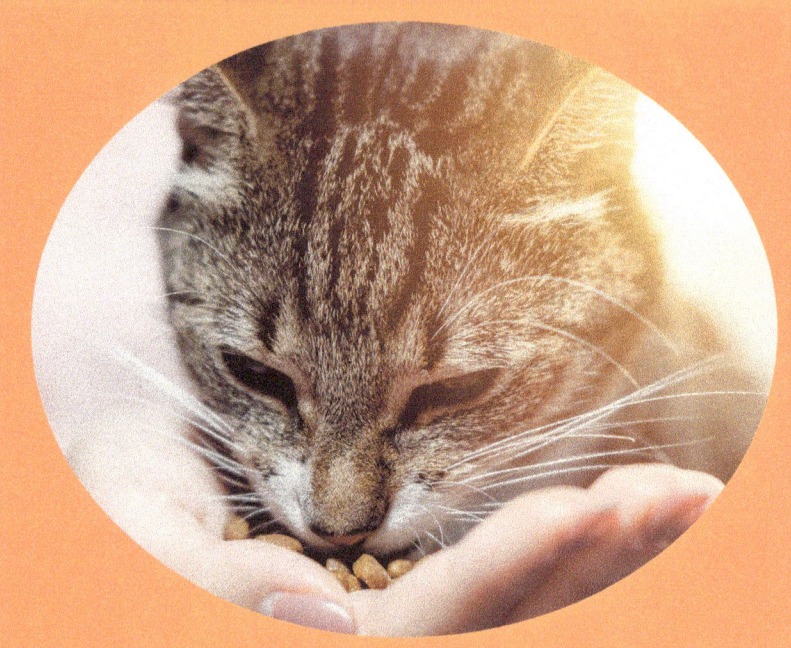

Before long, the kitten gets big and strong and doesn't need his mother's milk anymore.

He wants what big cats eat.

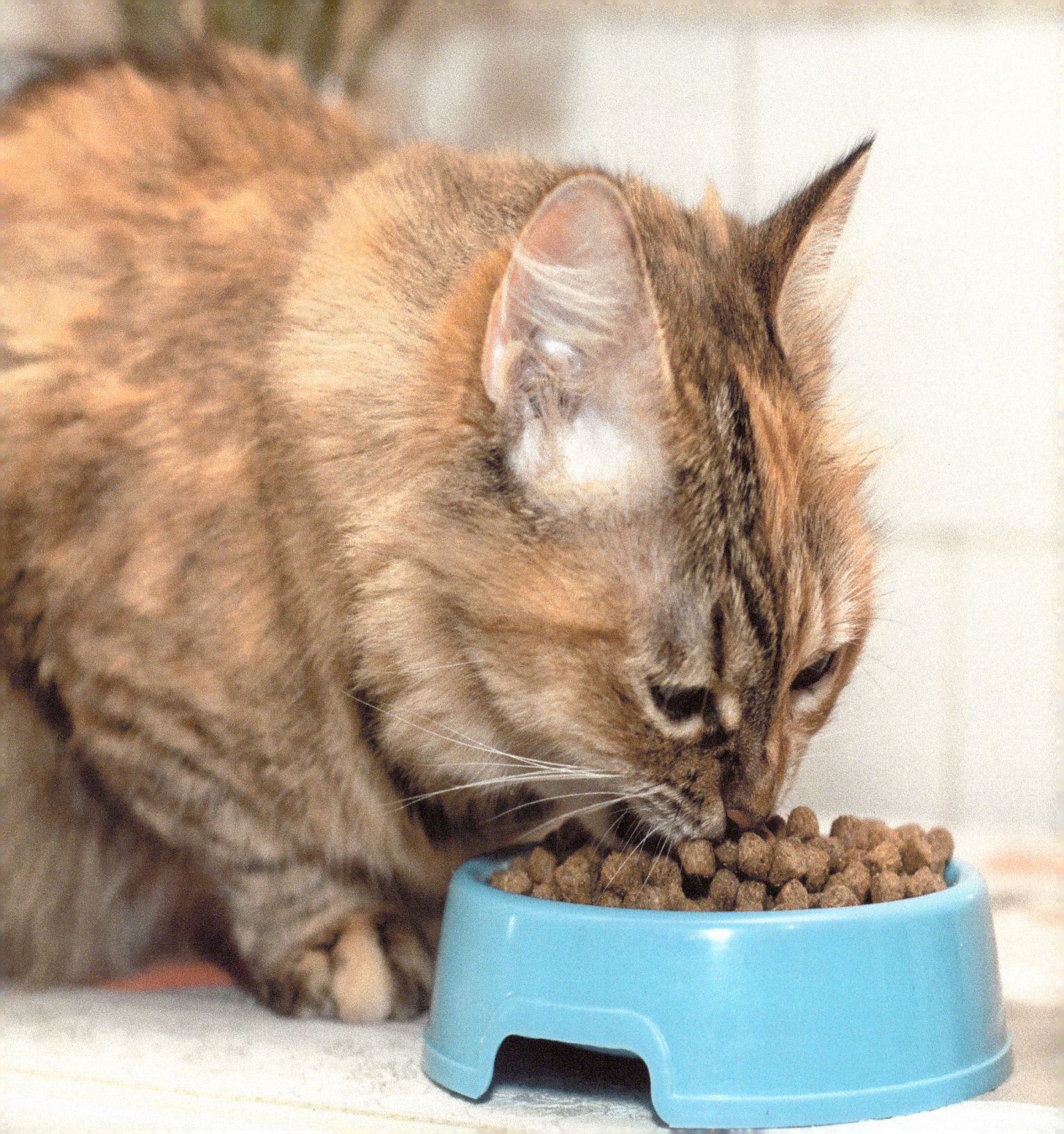

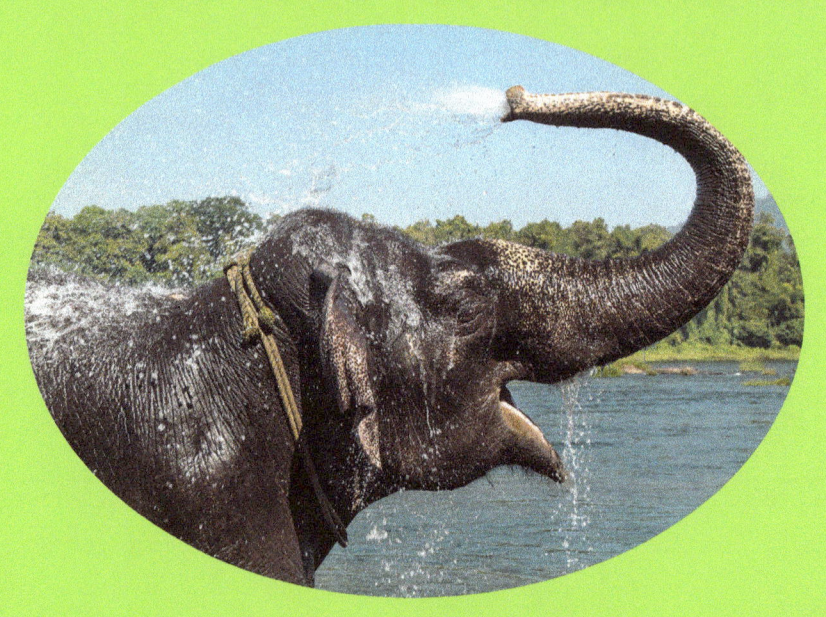

And here's a happy young elephant who loves to eat flowers and grasses.

His mother's milk made him strong so he doesn't need it now.

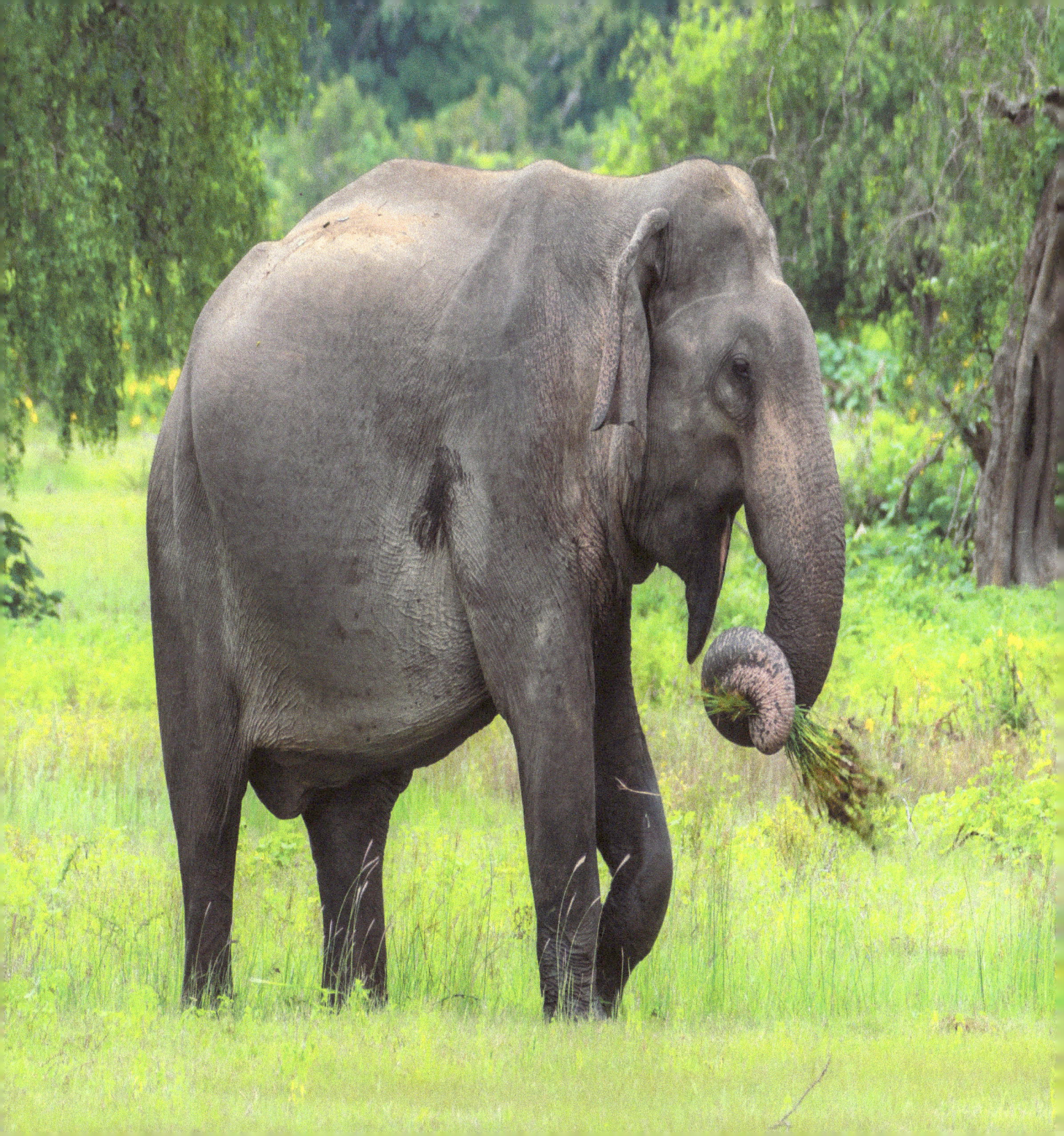

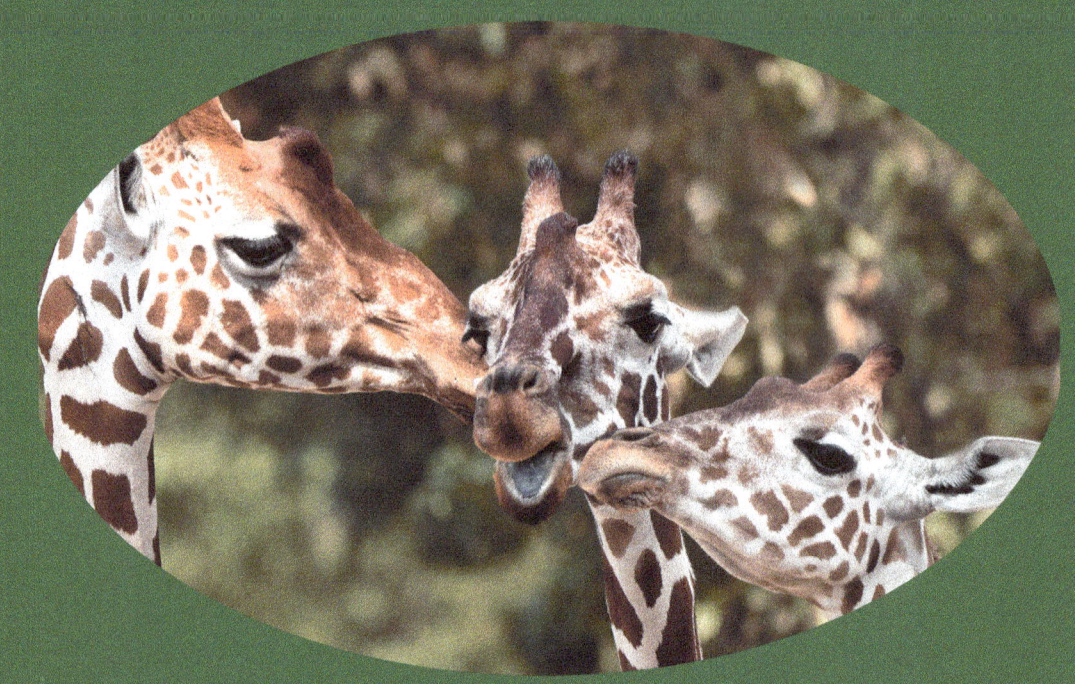

This pretty young giraffe is up on her long legs and stretching her long neck to get some tasty leaves from the tree tops.

She doesn't need mother's milk now.

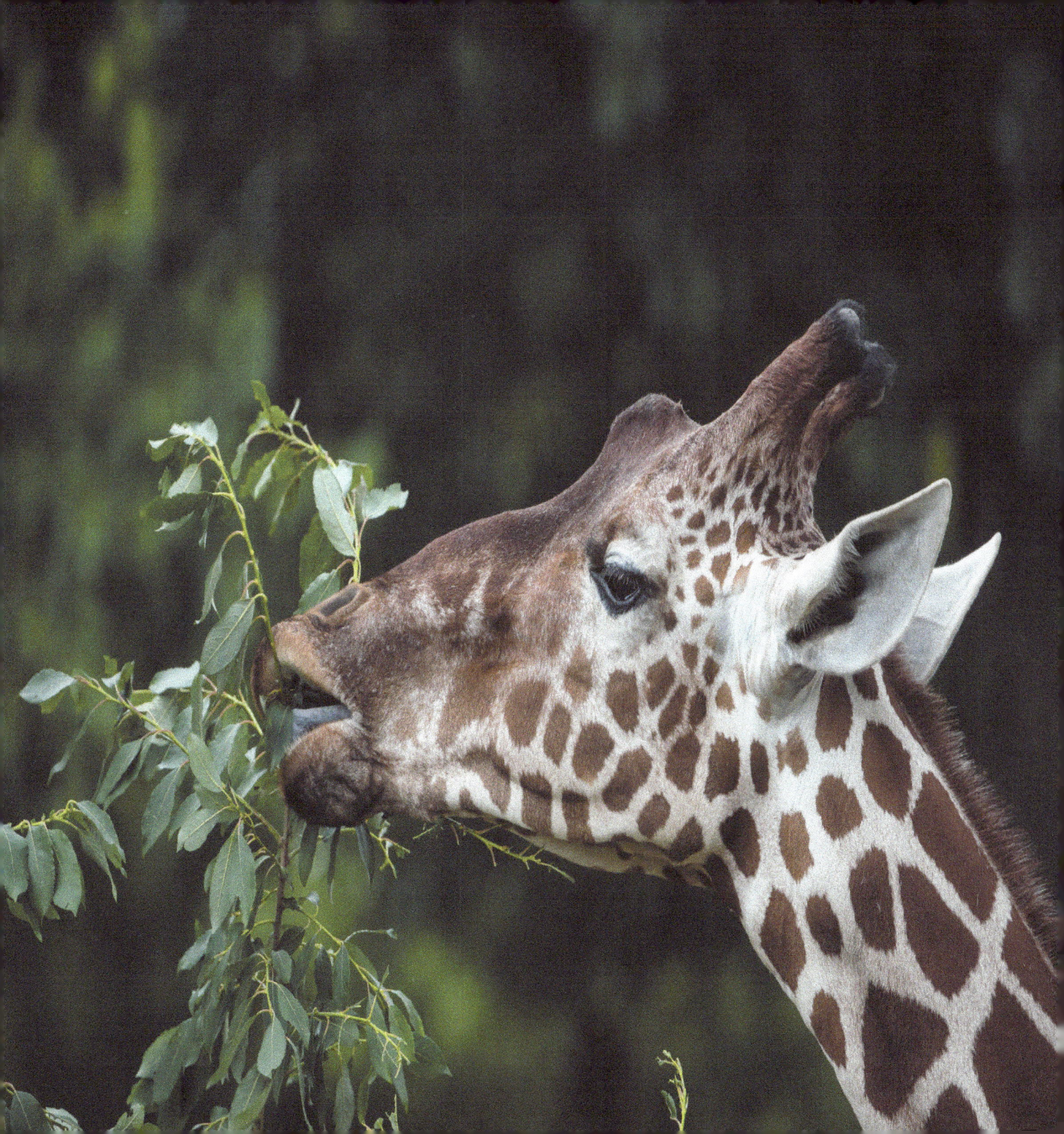

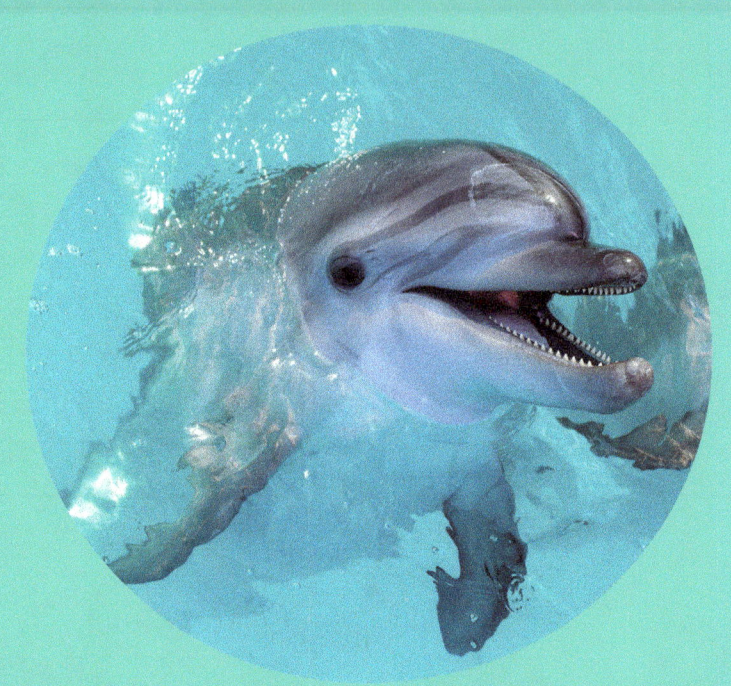

Here's a happy dolphin who grew big enough to catch and eat some tasty fish.

This guy won't be needing momma's milk.

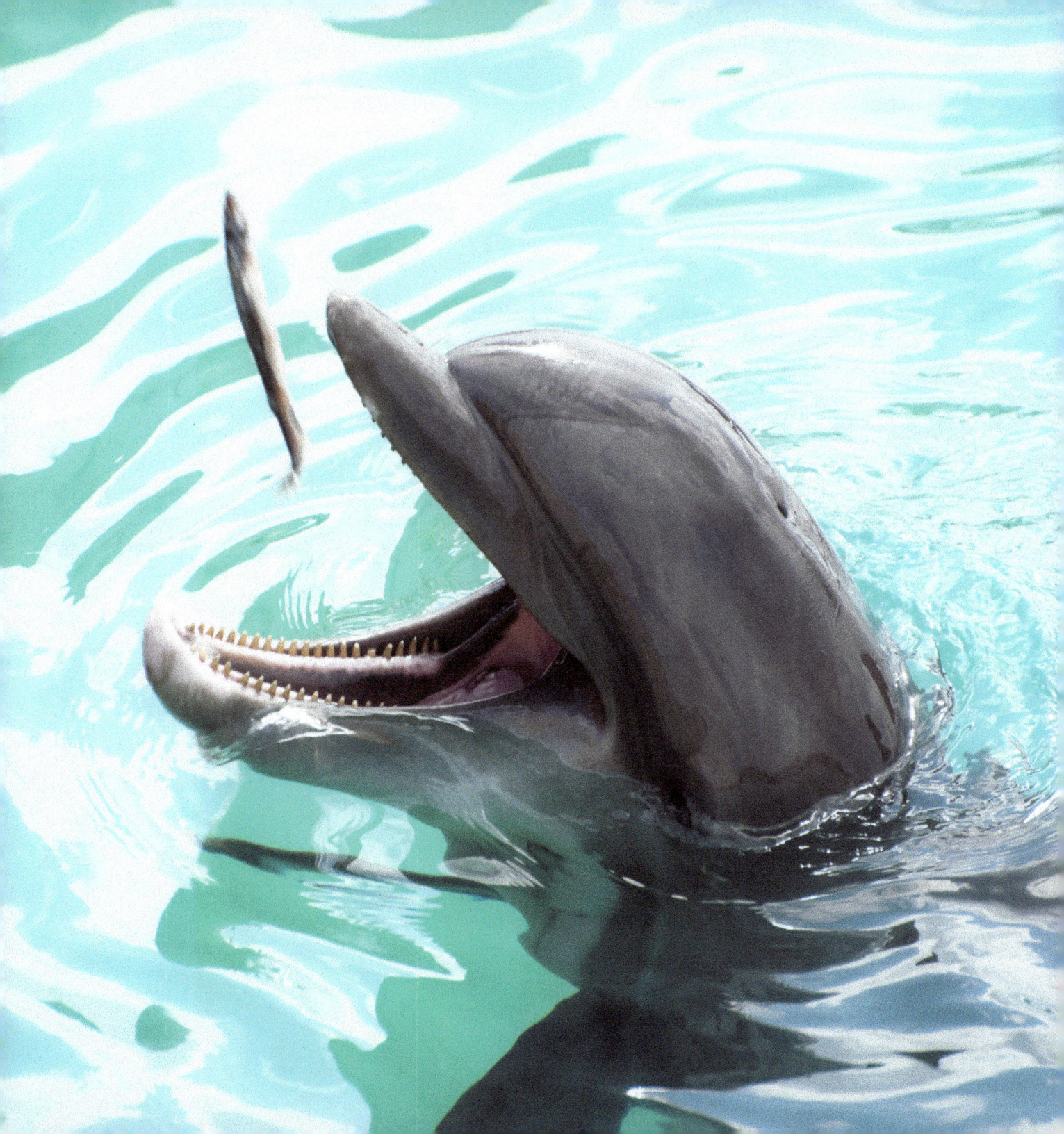

And when boys and girls grow up, they don't need milk from their mother any more either.

Big kids grow strong on fruits and vegetables and meat and grains.

All these foods make a kid's growing body strong.

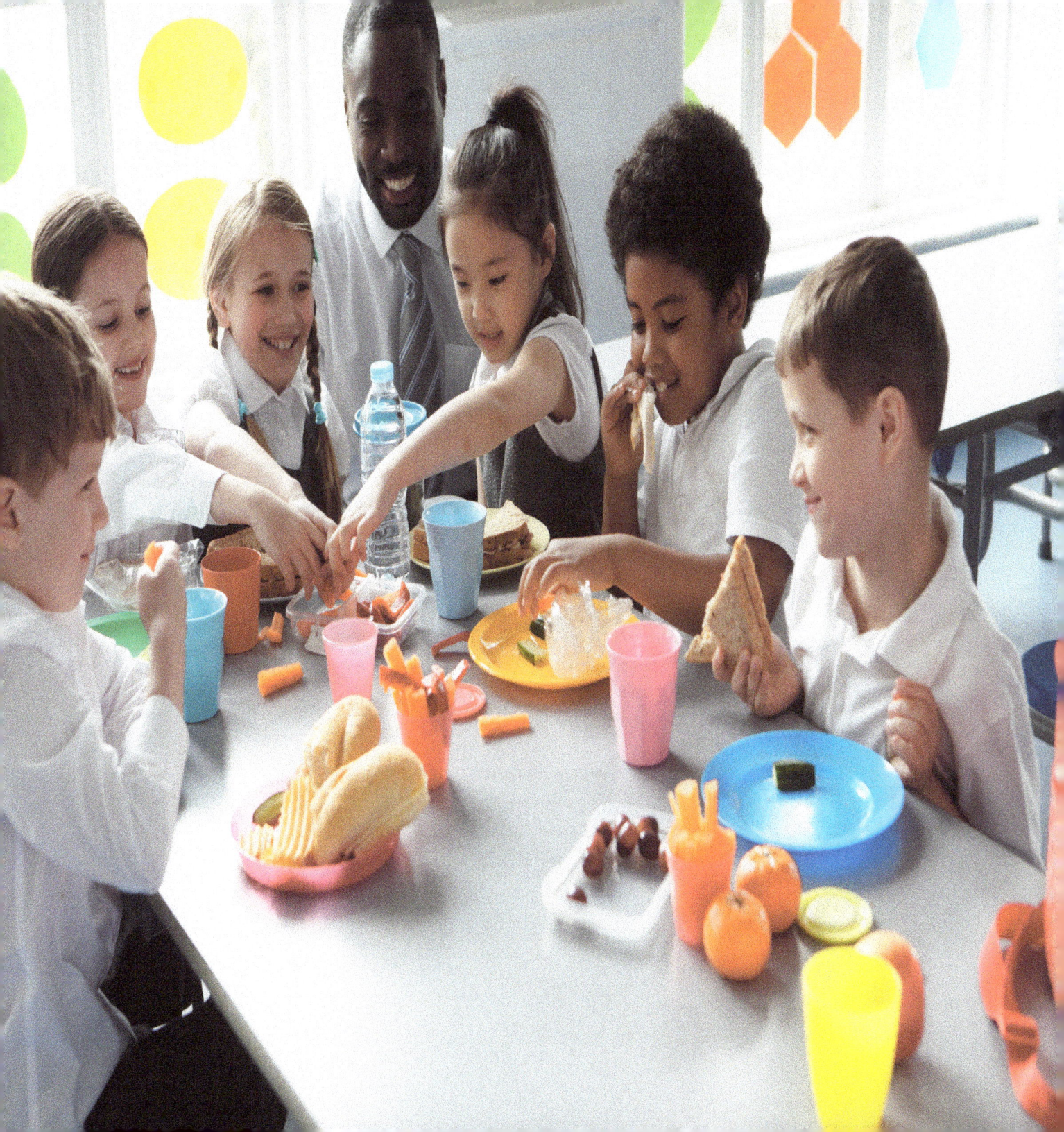

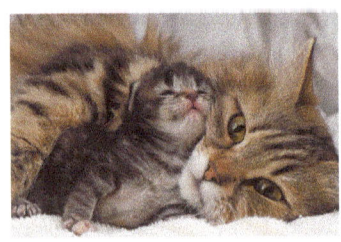
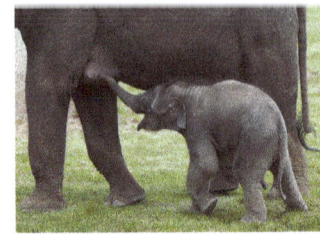
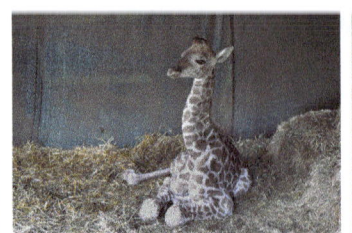
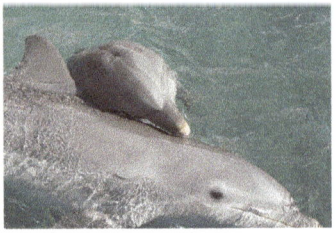
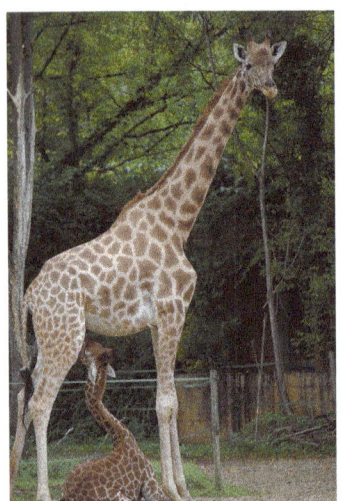
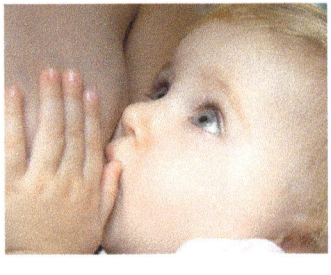
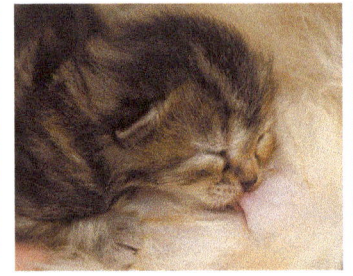
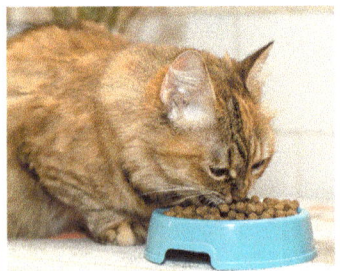
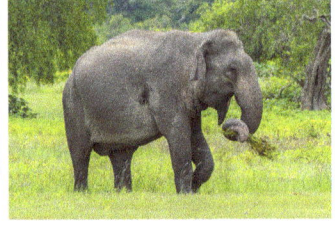
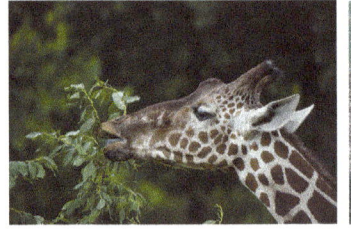
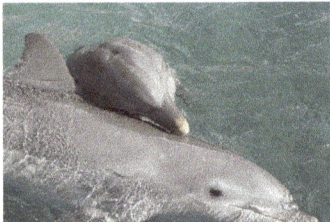
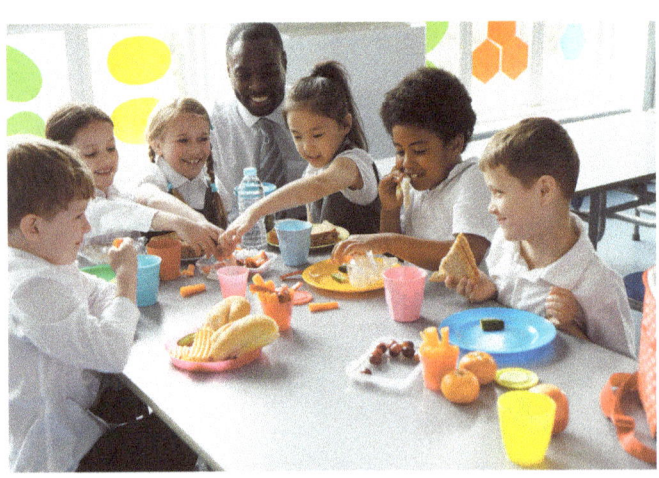
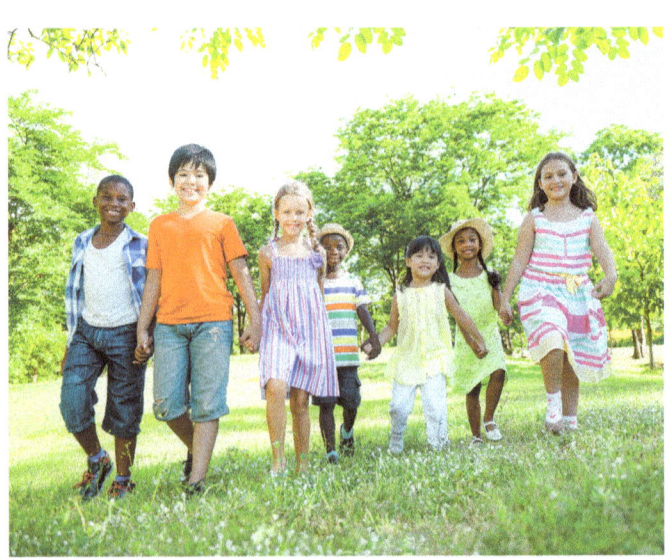

The End
of this book

and

The Beginning of many exciting
days to come...

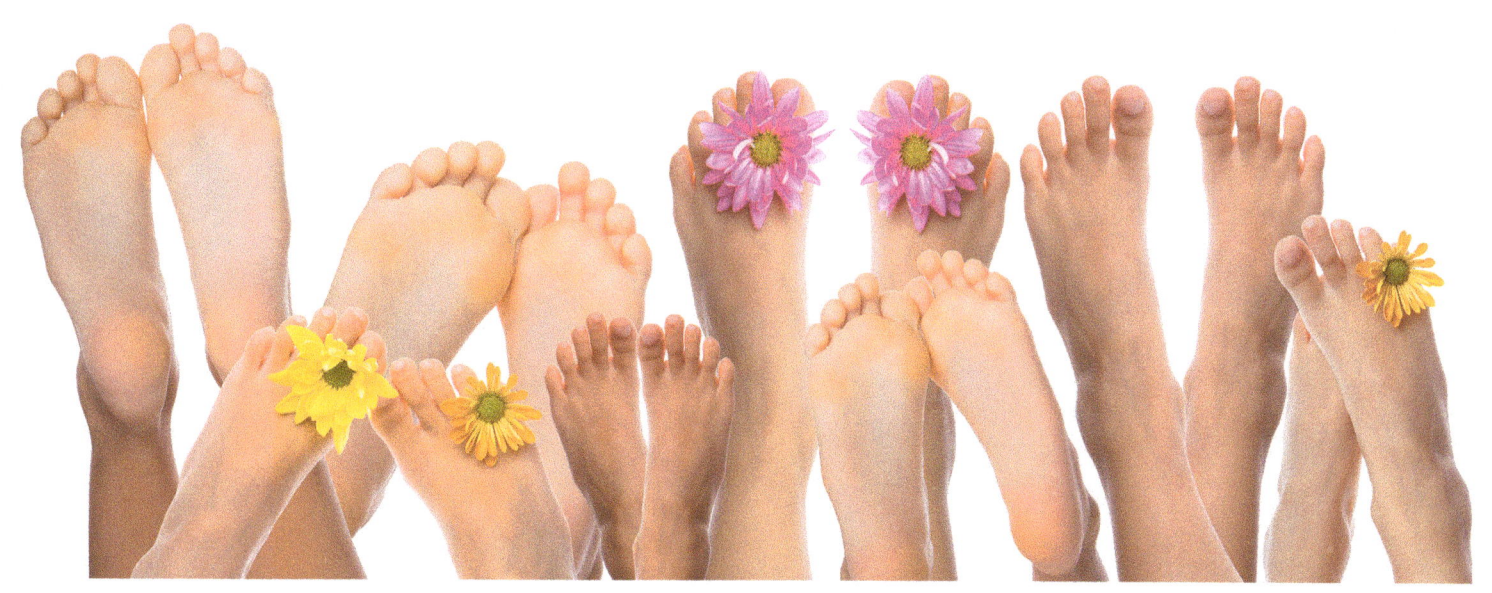

www.ingramcontent.com/pod-product-compliance
Lightning Source LLC
Chambersburg PA
CBHW040225040426
42333CB00054B/3452